MW00511012

Mastering The Air Fryer Grill

A Straightforward Guide To Learn How To Use The Air Fryer Grill And Enjoyable, Quick & Easy Recipes To Trigger All The Power Of Your Air Fryer Oven Grill And Appreciate With Your Family Healthy Food

Paty Breads

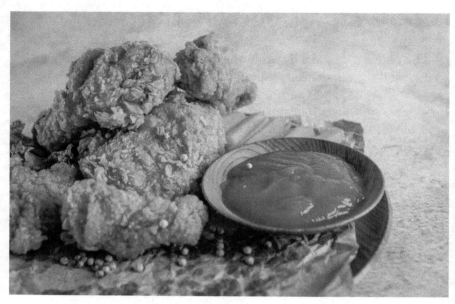

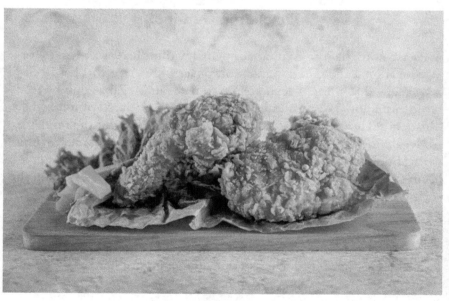

TABLE OF CONTENTS

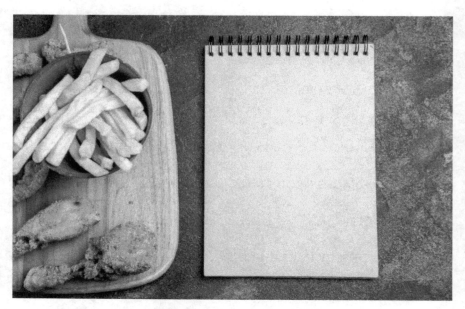

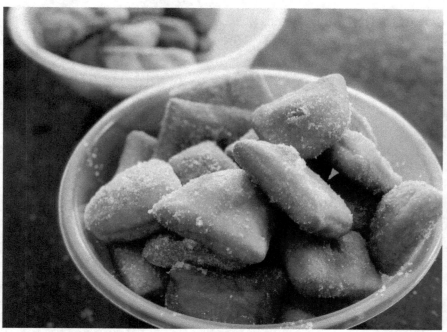

Introduction

The Power Air Fryer Grill may be a sophisticated machine imbued with modern technology for cooking healthy and luxurious meals quickly and as fast as possible. It's a multi-functional Air Fryer plus grill amid eight cook programs and intrinsic cooking presets. With the rapid air technology, heated air at 450°F circulates and cooks your meals 40% faster than ordinary/traditional cooking methods.

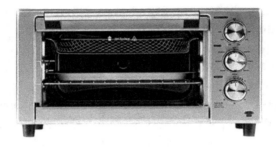

The Power Air Fryer Grill cuts calories in your meals by 70% due to the small quantity of oil required to grill, fry, and bake. It also saves time, counter space, and even the environment since it works via electricity.

Components and Functions of Power Air Fryer Grill

The Power Air Fryer Grill may be a box-like appliance comprising eight cooking/preset programs and straightforward work commands. The components and functions are as follows:

- The central unit may be a chrome steel construct that houses the component, instrument panel, and cooking accessories (pans, trays, and racks) through the three available tray ports.
- The tempered glass door keeps the warmth in and allows for even circulation of the recent air. Open and shut the door with the handle attached to avoid burns from the heated glass.
- The chrome steel drip tray placed below the component collects fluids and oils in cooking; if the drip tray is absent while cooking, it causes smoke and damaged heating coils.

- The grill plate is used to grill meat, burgers, vegetables, and more.
- The pizza rack is used to roast, toast bread & bagel, make pizza, and grill.
- The baking pan and the crisper tray are used to broil and make food without oil content.
- The instrument panel comprises knobs and buttons to regulate and adjust the time, temperature, and cooking programs. The preset programs are: air fry, grill, air fry/grill, rotisserie, toast/bagel, and pizza/bake, broil, and reheat.

How Power Air Fryer Grill Functions

- Set up your unit on a good, flat surface, preferably a cool countertop, far away from other appliances, and in a well-ventilated room. Plug the cord into a wall plug.
- Place the drip tray correctly at the unit's bottom and insert the proper accessory to make the food.
- Arrange the ingredients inside the unit.
- Select the specified cook program with the function knob.
- Select the temperature and time with the temperature/darkness control knob and, therefore, the time control knob. The facility light then comes on.
- The power light darkens, and the timer sounds once the cooking process ends. Note that foods cooked for fewer than 20 minutes don't activate the timer sound. Turn all knobs to the offsetting before opening the unit to get food.

Maintenance, Cleaning, and Tips

Proper and regular maintenance is crucial to machinery's long lifetime, and therefore the Power Air Fryer Grill isn't an exception.

- When unpacking for the first time, read all instructions and warnings, remove all labels, and wash all accessories with warm water and soap by hand. Preheat to reduce the producer's oil coat. Make sure you wipe off the melted oil with a moist rag before use.

- All accessories are dishwasher safe. Wash with soap and water. Most units must not be soaked or dipped in water but gently wiped inside and out first with a hot/soapy damp/soft rag then rinsed with a classic moist rag. Ensure it's completely dry before you turning it on.

- Wear protective gloves or oven mitts when handling any part of the Air Fryer grill to avoid burns.

- The Air Fryer grill is for indoor use only. Connect only to direct power sources, sort of wall plug, and never an extension box to avoid tripping accidents.

- The more the number of food, the longer it takes to cook and the other way around.

- You may use an oven dish or baking tin for filled foods like soups by placing it on the rack.

- Use parchment paper on the Air Fryer rack and drip pan to stop smoke as grease drops on the heating coils.

- Judiciously study the user manual of your appliance to stop eventualities and cure them.

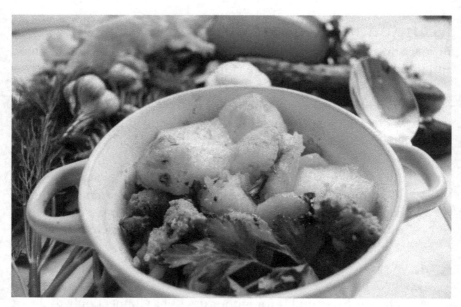

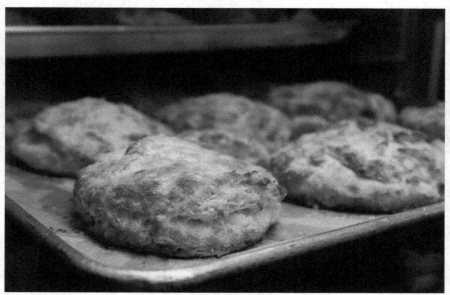

Chapter 1:

Breakfast Recipes

1. Brown Sugar Bacon Waffles

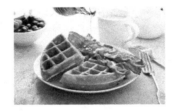

Preparation time: 18 minutes.

Cooking time: 25 minutes. **Servings:** 7

Ingredients:

- 7 slices bacon

- 3 cups flour

- 1 tablespoon baking powder

- 1 teaspoon baking soda and salt

- 1/2 cup brown sugar

- 4 eggs

- 2 teaspoons vanilla extract

- 2/3 cup grapeseed oil

- 2 cups buttermilk

Directions:

1. Incorporate all the dry ingredients and then wet ingredients to make the batter.

2. Preheat the Power Air Fryer Grill to 180°C or 350°F.

3. Grease the waffle pan, pour the mix, and bake for 15 minutes.

Nutrition:

- **Calories:** 389 **Protein:** 18.4g

- **Fat:** 23g

2. Italian Waffle Cookies

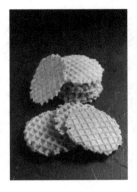

Preparation time: 19 minutes.

Cooking time: 12 minutes.

Servings: 4

Ingredients:

- 4 cups flour

- 1 cup butter

- 6 eggs

- 1 teaspoon vanilla extract

- 1–1/2 cup sugar

- 1/4 teaspoon salt

Directions:

1. Beat the eggs until thick. Mix in melted butter.

2. Mix the remaining ingredients to make the batter.

3. Preheat the Power Air Fryer Grill to 200°C or 400°F.

4. Bake the batter in a waffle pan for 15–18 minutes.

Nutrition:

- **Calories:** 132

- **Protein:** 2g

- **Fat:** 5g

3. Strawberry Ricotta Waffles

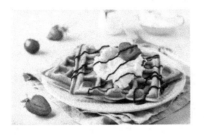

Preparation time: 8 minutes.

Cooking time: 12 minutes.

Servings: 2

Ingredients:

- 2 cups flour

- 1 teaspoon baking soda

- 2 eggs

- 2 tablespoons sugar

- 1/2 teaspoons vanilla extract

- 2 cups milk

- 1/4 cup oil

- 1/2 cup strawberries, sliced

- 1/4 cup ricotta cheese

- 2 teaspoons maple syrup

Directions:

1. Preheat the Power Air Fryer Grill to 200°C or 400°F.

2. Whisk the dry and wet batter ingredients.

3. Fill in the batter into the mold and bake for 12–15 minutes.

4. Mix ricotta and vanilla in a bowl. Top with the mixture, syrup, and strawberries.

Nutrition:

- **Calories:** 318

- **Protein:** 11.9g

- **Fat:** 13.6g

4. Pineapple Bagel Brulee

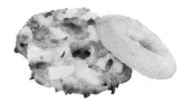

Preparation time: 6 minutes.

Cooking time: 15 minutes.

Servings: 8

Ingredients:

- 4 thin bagels

- 4 teaspoons brown sugar

- 3/4 cup low-fat cream cheese

- 8 slices pineapples

- 3 tablespoons almonds, toasted

Directions:

1. Preheat the Power Air Fryer Grill to 220°C or 425°F.

2. Bake the pineapple slices with brown sugar sprinkled on top.

3. Toast bagels and apply cream cheese, almonds, and baked pineapples.

Nutrition:

- **Calories:** 157

- **Protein:** 5.6g

- **Fat:** 6.4g

5. Golden Egg Bagels

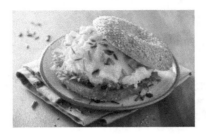

Preparation time: 4 minutes.

Cooking time: 16 minutes.

Servings: 8

Ingredients:

- 2 eggs

- 4 teaspoons dry yeast 4–5 cups all-purpose flour

- 1 tablespoon canola oil and kosher salt

- 1–1/2 tablespoon sugar

Directions:

1. Whisk eggs, sugar, yeast, lukewarm, water, and oil. Add flour
   and salt to prepare the dough.

2. Make a long rope with the dough, locking both ends.

3. Preheat the Power Air Fryer Grill to 200°C or 400°F.

4. Boil bagels in sugar and salt for 45 seconds.

5. Drain bagels, brush with egg white, and bake for 15–20 minutes.

Nutrition:

- **Calories:** 164

- **Protein:** 6.6g

- **Fat:** 2.1g

6. Spinach Egg Breakfast

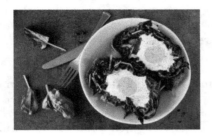

Preparation time: 10 minutes.

Cooking time: 20 minutes.

Servings: 4

Ingredients:

- 3 eggs

- 1/4 cup coconut milk

- 1/4 cup Parmesan cheese, grated

- 4 ounces spinach, chopped

- 3 ounces Cottage cheese

Directions:

1. Preheat the Air Fryer to 350°F.

2. Add eggs, milk, half Parmesan cheese, and Cottage cheese in a

   bowl and whisk well. Add spinach and stir well.

3. Pour mixture into the Air Fryer baking dish.

4. Sprinkle remaining half Parmesan cheese on top.

5. Put it in the Air Fryer, then cook for 20 minutes.

6. Serve and enjoy!

Nutrition:

- **Calories:** 144

- **Fat:** 8.5g

- **Carbohydrates:** 2.5 g

- **Sugar:** 1.1g

- **Protein:** 14g

- **Cholesterol:** 135mg

7. Vegetable Quiche

Preparation time: 10 minutes.

Cooking time: 24 minutes.

Servings: 6

Ingredients:

- 8 eggs

- 1 cup of coconut milk

- 1 cup tomatoes, chopped

- 1 cup zucchini, chopped

- 1 tablespoon butter

- 1 onion, chopped

- 1 cup Parmesan cheese, grated

- 1/2 teaspoon pepper

- 1 teaspoon salt

Directions:

1. Preheat the Air Fryer to 370°F.

2. Melt butter in a pan, then add onion and sauté until onion is

    lightly brown.

3. Add tomatoes and zucchini to the pan and sauté for 4–5 minutes.

4. Transfer cooked vegetables into the Air Fryer baking dish.

5. Beat eggs with cheese, milk, pepper, and salt in a bowl.

6. Pour egg mixture over vegetables in a baking dish.

7. Put it in the Air Fryer, then cook for 24 minutes or until eggs

    are set.

8. Slice and serve.

Nutrition:

- **Calories:** 255 **Fat:** 16g

- **Carbohydrates:** 8g **Sugar:** 4.2g

- **Protein:** 21g

- **Cholesterol:** 257mg

Chapter 2:

Meat Recipes

8. Coffee Flavored Steak

Preparation time: 10 minutes.

Cooking time: 15 minutes.

Servings: 4

Ingredients:

- 4 rib-eye steak

- 2 tablespoons garlic powder

- 2 tablespoons chili powder

- 1–1/2 tablespoon ground coffee

- 2 tablespoons onion powder

- 1/2 tablespoon sweet paprika

- Pinch of cayenne pepper

- 1/4 teaspoon ground ginger

- Black pepper to taste

- 1/4 teaspoon ground coriander

Directions:

1. Preheat the Air Fryer to 360°F.

2. In a bowl, mix all the ingredients excluding the steak, and stir.

   Rub the steak thoroughly with the mixture.

3. Transfer to the Air Fryer and cook for 15 minutes.

4. Serve and enjoy!

Nutrition:

- **Calories:** 160 **Fat:** 10g **Carb:** 14g

- **Proteins:** 12g

9. Seasoned Beef Roast

Preparation time: 10 minutes.

Cooking time: 45 minutes.

Servings: 10

Ingredients:

- 3 pounds beef top roast

- 1 tablespoon olive oil

- 2 tablespoons Montreal steak seasoning

Directions:

1. Coat the roast with oil and then rub with the seasoning generously.

2. With kitchen twines, tie the roast to keep it compact. Arrange the roast onto the cooking tray.

3. Select "Air Fry" and then alter the temperature to 360°F. Set the timer for 45 minutes and press the "Start."

4. If the display shows "Add Food," insert the cooking tray in the center position.

5. When the display shows "Turn Food," do nothing.

6. When cooking time is completed, take away the tray from Vortex.

7. Place the roast onto a platter for about 10 minutes before slicing.

8. With a sharp knife, cut the roast into desired-sized slices and serve.

Nutrition:

- **Calories:** 269

- **Fat:** 9.9g

- **Carbs:** 0g

- **Fiber:** 0g

10. Simple Beef Sirloin Roast

Preparation time: 10 minutes.

Cooking time: 50 minutes.

Servings: 8

Ingredients:

- 2(½) pounds sirloin roast

- Salt and ground black pepper, as required

Directions:

1. Rub the roast with salt and black pepper generously.

2. Insert the rotisserie rod through the roast.

3. Insert the rotisserie forks, one on each rod's side, to secure the rod to the chicken.

4. Select "Roast" and then adjust the temperature to 350°F.

5. Set the timer for 50 minutes and press the "Start."

6. When the display shows "Add Food," press the red lever down.

7. Weight the left side of the rod into the Vortex.

8. Now, turn the rod's left side into the groove along the metal bar so it will not move.

9. Then, close the door and touch "Rotate." Press the red lever to release the rod when cooking time is completed.

10. Remove from the Vortex.

11. Place the roast onto a platter for about 10 minutes before slicing.

12. With a sharp knife, cut the roast into desired-sized slices and serve.

Nutrition:

- **Calories:** 201

- **Fat:** 8.8g

- **Carbs:** 0g

- **Protein:** 28.9g

11. Simple Beef Patties

Preparation time: 10 minutes.

Cooking time: 13 minutes.

Servings: 4

Ingredients:

- 1-pound ground beef

- ½ teaspoon garlic powder

- ¼ teaspoon onion powder

- Pepper to taste

- Salt to taste

Directions:

1. Preheat the instant vortex Air Fryer oven to 400°F.

2. Add ground meat, garlic powder, onion powder, pepper, and

   salt into the mixing bowl and mix until well combined.

3. Make even shape patties from the meat mixture and arrange them on an Air Fryer pan.

4. Place pan in the instant vortex, Air Fryer oven.

5. Cook patties for 10 minutes. Turn patties after 5 minutes

6. Serve and enjoy!

Nutrition:

- **Calories:** 212

- **Fat:** 7.1g

- **Carbs:** 0.4g

- **Protein:** 34.5g

12. Beef Sirloin Roast

Preparation time: 10 minutes.

Cooking time: 50 minutes.

Servings: 8

Ingredients:

- 1 tablespoon smoked paprika

- 1 teaspoon ground cumin

- 1 teaspoon garlic powder

- Salt and freshly ground black pepper to taste

- 2(½) pounds sirloin roast

Directions:

1. In a bowl, mix together the spices, salt, and black pepper.

2. Rub the roast with spice mixture generously.

3. Place the sirloin roast into the greased baking pan.

4. Press the "Power Button" of Power Digital Air Fry oven and turn the dial to select "Air Roast" mode.

5. Press the "Time Button" and again turn the dial to set the cooking time to 50 minutes.

6. Now push "Temp Button" and rotate the dial to set the temperature to 350°F.

7. Press the "Start/Pause" button to start.

8. When the unit beeps to show that it is preheated, open the lid and insert the baking pan in the oven.

9. When cooking time is completed, open the lid and place the roast onto a platter for about 10 minutes before slicing.

10. With a sharp knife, cut the beef roast into desired-sized slices and serve.

Nutrition:

- **Calories:** 260 **Fat:** 11.9g **Carbohydrates:** 0.4g **Fiber:** 0.1g

- **Sugar:** 0.1g **Protein:** 38g

13. Air Fried Grilled Steak

Preparation time: 6 minutes.

Cooking time: 40 minutes.

Servings: 2

Ingredients:

- 2 sirloin steaks

- 3 tablespoons butter, melted

- 3 tablespoons olive oil

- Salt and pepper to taste

Directions:

1. Preheat the Power Air Fryer Grill for 5 minutes to 350°F.

2. Season the sirloin steaks with olive oil, salt, and pepper.

3. Place the beef in the Air Fryer basket and put the basket into the oven.

4. Select grill. Grill for 40 minutes at 350°F.

5. Once cooked, serve with butter.

Nutrition:

- **Calories:** 1536

- **Fat:** 123.7g

- **Protein:** 103.4g

14. Air Fryer Beef Casserole

Preparation time: 7 minutes.

Cooking time: 30 minutes.

Servings: 4

Ingredients:

- 1 green bell pepper, seeded and chopped

- 1 onion, chopped

- 1-pound ground beef

- 3 garlic cloves, minced

- 6 cups eggs, beaten

Directions:

1. Preheat the Air Fryer for 5 minutes to 325°F.

2. In a baking dish, mix the ground beef, onion, garlic, olive oil, and bell pepper.

3. Add beaten eggs to a large bowl.

4. Season the ground beef mixture with salt and pepper and pour in the beaten eggs and give a good stir.

5. Place the dish with the beef and egg mixture in the Air Fryer.

6. Place the rack on the middle shelf of the Air Fryer.

7. Select bake. Set temperature to 325°F and set time to 30 minutes.

8. When done, remove from the oven and rest for 5 minutes. Serve warm.

Nutrition:

- **Calories:** 1520

- **Fat:** 125.1g

- **Protein:** 87.9g

15. Charred Onions & Steak Cube BBQ

Preparation time: 8 minutes.

Cooking time: 40 minutes.

Servings: 3

Ingredients:

- 1 cup red onions, cut into wedges

- 1 tablespoon dry mustard

- 1 tablespoon olive oil

- 1-pound boneless beef sirloin, cut into cubes

- Salt and pepper to taste

Directions:

1. Preheat the Air Fryer to 390°F.

2. Place the grill rack in the Air Fryer. Toss all the listed ingredients in a bowl and mix until everything is coated with the seasonings.

3. Place on the grill rack and put the rack in the oven.

4. Select grill. Grill for 40 minutes.

5. Halfway through the cooking time, give a stir to cook evenly.

6. When done, transfer to a plate and enjoy!

Nutrition:

- **Calories:** 260

- **Fat:** 10.7g

- **Protein:** 35.5g

16. Beef Ribeye Steak

Preparation time: 6 minutes.

Cooking time: 10 minutes.

Servings: 4

Ingredients:

- 4 (8-ounces) rib-eye steaks

- 1 tablespoon McCormick Grill Mates Montreal Steak Seasoning

- Salt and pepper to taste

Directions:

1. Season the steaks with salt, pepper, and seasoning.

2. Place two steaks in the Power Air Fryer Grill rack.

3. Select grill and grill for 5 minutes at 400°F.

4. Open the Air Fryer and flip the steaks. Then cook for an additional 5 minutes.

5. Remove the cooked steaks from the Power Air Fryer Grill to a

   plate.

6. Repeat for the remaining two steaks.

7. Serve warm.

Nutrition:

- **Calories:** 293

- **Fat:** 22g

- **Fiber:** 0g

- **Protein:** 23g

Chapter 3:

Poultry Recipes

17. Paprika Chicken Wings

Preparation time: 15 minutes.

Cooking time: 24 minutes.

Servings: 6

Ingredients:

- 1(½) pound chicken wings

- 1/4 teaspoon sea salt

- 1/2 teaspoon black pepper

- 1/2 teaspoon smoked paprika

- 1/2 teaspoon garlic powder

- 1/2 teaspoon baking powder

- 1/2 teaspoon onion powder

Directions:

1. Mix smoked paprika, black pepper, salt, garlic powder, baking powder, and onion powder in a small bowl.

2. Add all the chicken wings to a large bowl and drizzle the spice mixture over the wings.

3. Toss well and transfer the wings to an Air Fryer basket.

4. Return the Air Fryer basket to the Air Fryer.

5. Select the Air Fry mode at 400°F for 24 minutes.

6. Toss the wings once cooked halfway through.

7. Serve warm.

Nutrition:

- **Calories:** 220 **Fat:** 1.7g **Sodium:** 178mg **Carbs:** 1.7g

- **Fiber:** 0.2g **Sugar:** 0.2g **Protein:** 32.9g

18. Breaded Chicken Legs

Preparation time: 20 minutes.

Cooking time: 24 minutes.

Servings: 6

Ingredients:

- 12 chicken legs

- 2 tablespoons seasoned salt

- 4 tablespoons olive oil

- 1 bag of chicken breading

Directions:

1. Toss drumsticks with olive oil and drizzle seasoning on top

2. Mix well to coat and coat the drumsticks with breadcrumbs.

3. Place the coated drumsticks in the Air Fryer basket and spray them with cooking oil.

4. Return the Air Fryer basket to the Air Fryer.

5. Select the Air Fry mode at 400°F for 24 minutes.

6. Flip the drumsticks once cooked halfway through, then resume cooking.

7. Serve warm.

Nutrition:

- **Calories:** 380

- **Fat:** 29g

- **Sodium:** 821mg

- **Carbs:** 34.6g

- **Fiber:** 0g

- **Sugar:** 0g

- **Protein:** 30g

19. Herbed Chicken Breast

Preparation time: 15 minutes.

Cooking time: 22 minutes.

Servings: 4

Ingredients:

- 4 boneless, skinless chicken breasts

- 1/2 teaspoon garlic powder

- 1/2 teaspoon salt

- 1/8 teaspoon black pepper

- 1/2 teaspoon dried oregano

Directions:

1. Mix garlic powder, oregano, black pepper, and salt in a small

   bowl.

2. Spray the chicken breast with cooking spray.

3. Rub the chicken with the seasoning mix liberally.

4. Place the seasoned chicken breast in the Air Fryer basket.

5. Return the Air Fryer basket to the Air Fryer.

6. Select the air fry mode at 360°F for 22 minutes.

7. Flip the chicken once cooked halfway through, drizzle the remaining seasoning.

8. Resume cooking and cook until the chicken is golden.

9. Serve warm.

Nutrition:

- **Calories:** 268

- **Fat:** 10.4g **Sodium:** 411mg

- **Carbs:** 0.4g

- **Fiber:** 0.1g

- **Sugar:** 0.1g

- **Protein:** 40.6g

20. Chicken with Asparagus, Beans, and

Arugula

Preparation time: 20 minutes.

Cooking time: 25 minutes. **Servings:** 2

Ingredients:

- 1 cup canned cannellini beans, rinsed

- 1(½) tablespoons red wine vinegar

- 1 garlic clove, minced

- 2 tablespoons extra-virgin olive oil, divided

- Salt and ground black pepper to taste

- ½ red onion, sliced thinly

- 8 ounces (227 grams) asparagus, trimmed and cut into 1-inch

  lengths

- 2 (8-ounces/227 grams) boneless, skinless chicken breasts,

  trimmed

- ¼ teaspoon paprika

- ½ teaspoon ground coriander

- 2 ounces (57 grams) baby arugula, rinsed and drained

Directions:

1. Warm the beans in the microwave for 1 minute and combine with red wine vinegar, garlic, 1 tablespoon of olive oil, ¼ teaspoon of salt, and ¼ teaspoon of ground black pepper in a bowl. Stir to mix well.

2. Combine the onion with 1/8 teaspoon of salt, 1/8 teaspoon of ground black pepper, and 2 teaspoons of olive oil in a separate bowl. Toss to coat well.

3. Place the onion in the airflow racks.

4. Slide the racks into the Air Fryer oven. Press the power button. Cook at 400°F (205°C) for 2 minutes.

5. After 2 minutes, add the asparagus for 8 minutes. Stir the vegetable halfway through.

6. When cooking is completed, the asparagus should be tender.

7. Transfer the onion and asparagus to the bowl with beans. Set aside.

8. Toss the chicken breasts with the remaining ingredients, except for the baby arugula, in a large bowl.

9. Put the chicken breasts in the airflow racks. Slide the racks into the Air Fryer oven. Cook for 14 minutes. Flip the breasts halfway through.

10. When cooking is completed, the internal temperature of the chicken reaches at least 165°F (74°C).

11. Remove the chicken from the Air Fryer oven and serve on an aluminum foil with asparagus, beans, onion, and arugula. Sprinkle with salt and ground black pepper. Toss to serve.

Nutrition

- **Calories:** 166 **Protein:** 19g

- **Fat:** 9g

21. Chicken with Potatoes and Corn

Preparation time: 10 minutes.**Cooking time:** 25 minutes.

Servings: 4

Ingredients:

- 4 bone-in, skin-on chicken thighs

- 2 teaspoons kosher salt, divided

- 1 cup Bisquick baking mix

- ½ cup butter, melted, divided

- 1 pound (454 grams) small red potatoes, quartered

- 3 ears corn, shucked and cut into rounds 1 to 1½-inches thick

- 1/3 cup heavy whipping cream

- ½ teaspoon freshly ground black pepper

Directions:

1. Season the chicken on all sides with 1 teaspoon of kosher salt.

   Place the baking mix in a shallow dish. Brush the thighs on all sides with ¼ cup of butter, then dredge them in the baking mix, coating them all on sides. Place the chicken in the center of a baking pan.

2. Place the potatoes in a large bowl with 2 tablespoons of butter and toss to coat. Place them on one side of the chicken on the pan.

3. Place the corn in a medium bowl and drizzle with the remaining butter. Sprinkle with ¼ teaspoon of kosher salt and toss to coat. Place on the pan on the other side of the chicken.

4. Slide the pan into the Air Fryer oven. Press the power button. Cook at 375°F (190°C) for 25 minutes.

5. After 20 minutes, remove from the Air Fryer oven and transfer the potatoes back to the bowl. Return the pan to the Air Fryer oven and continue cooking.

6. As the chicken continues cooking, add the cream, black pepper, and the remaining kosher salt to the potatoes. Lightly crush the potatoes with a potato masher.

7. When cooking is completed, the corn should be tender, and the chicken cooked through, reading 165°F (74°C) on a meat thermometer. Pull out the pan from the Air Fryer oven and serve the chicken with the mashed potatoes and corn on the side.

Nutrition:

- **Calories:** 199

- **Protein:** 24g

- **Fat:** 6g

22. China Spicy Turkey Thighs

Preparation time: 10 minutes.

Cooking time: 25 minutes.

Servings: 6

Ingredients:

- 2 pounds (907 grams) turkey thighs

- 1 teaspoon Chinese five-spice powder

- ¼ teaspoon Sichuan pepper

- 1 teaspoon pink Himalayan salt

- 1 tablespoon Chinese rice vinegar

- 1 tablespoon mustard

- 1 tablespoon chili sauce

- 2 tablespoons soy sauce Cooking spray for greasing

Directions:

1. Spray the airflow racks with cooking spray.

2. Rub the turkey thighs with five-spice powder, Sichuan pepper, and salt on a clean work surface.

3. Put the turkey thighs in the airflow racks and spray with cooking spray.

4. Slide the racks into the Air Fryer oven. Press the power button. Cook at 360°F (182°C) for 22 minutes.

5. Flip the thighs at least three times during the cooking.

6. When cooking is completed, the thighs should be well browned.

7. Meanwhile, heat the remaining ingredients in a saucepan over medium-high heat. Cook for 3 minutes or until the sauce is thickened and reduces to two-thirds.

8. Transfer the thighs onto a plate and baste with sauce before serving.

Nutrition:

- **Calories:** 194 **Protein:** 19g **Fat:** 6g

23. Creole Hens

Preparation time: 10 minutes.

Cooking time: 40 minutes.

Servings: 4

Ingredients:

- ½ tablespoon Creole seasoning

- ½ tablespoon garlic powder

- ½ tablespoon onion powder

- ½ tablespoons freshly ground black pepper

- ½ tablespoon paprika

- 2 tablespoons olive oil

- 2 Cornish hens

- Cooking spray for greasing

Directions:

1. Spray the airflow racks with cooking spray.

2. In a small bowl, mix the Creole seasoning, garlic powder, onion powder, pepper, and paprika.

3. Pat the Cornish hens dry and brush each hen all over with olive oil. Rub each hen with the seasoning mixture. Place the Cornish hens in the airflow racks.

4. Press the Power Button. Cook at 375°F (190°C) for 30 minutes.

5. After 15 minutes, remove from the Air Fryer oven. Flip the hens over and baste them with any drippings collected in the drip tray placed at the bottom of the Air Fryer oven. Return to the Air Fryer oven and continue cooking.

6. When cooking is completed, a thermometer inserted into the thickest part of the hens should reach at least 165°F (74°C).

7. Set aside for 10 minutes before carving.

Nutrition:

- **Calories:** 144 **Protein:** 19g **Fat:** 9g

24. Crispy Chicken Skin

Preparation time: 5 minutes.

Cooking time: 6 minutes.

Servings: 4

Ingredients:

- 1-pound (454 grams) chicken skin, cut into slices

- 1 teaspoon melted butter

- ½ teaspoon crushed chili flakes

- 1 teaspoon dried dill

- Salt and ground black pepper to taste

Directions:

1. Incorporate all the ingredients. Toss to coat the chicken skin

   well.

2. Transfer the skin to the airflow racks.

3. Slide the racks into the Air Fryer oven. Press the power button.

   Cook at 360°F (182°C) for 6 minutes.

4. Stir the skin halfway through.

5. When cooking is completed, the skin should be crispy.

6. Serve immediately.

Nutrition:

- **Calories:** 179

- **Protein:** 16g

- **Fat:** 6.7g

Chapter 4:

Vegetables Recipes

25. Roasted Squash

Preparation time: 10 minutes.

Cooking time: 35 minutes.

Servings: 6

Ingredients:

- 4 cups butternut squash, diced

- 1/4 cup dried cranberries

- 3 garlic cloves, minced

- 1 tablespoon soy sauce

- 1 tablespoon balsamic vinegar

- 1 tablespoon olive oil

- 8 ounces mushrooms, quartered

- 1 cup green onions, sliced

Directions:

1. In a large mixing bowl, blend squash, mushrooms, and green onion, and set aside.

2. In a small bowl, whisk together oil, garlic, vinegar, and soy sauce.

3. Pour oil mixture over squash and toss to coat.

4. Spray Air Fryer basket with cooking spray.

5. Add squash mixture into the Air Fryer basket and cook for 30–35 minutes at 400°F. Shake after every 5 minutes.

6. Toss with cranberries and serve hot.

Nutrition:

- **Calories:** 82 **Fat:** 2.6g **Carbohydrates:** 14.5g **Sugar:** 3.3g

- **Protein:** 2.7g **Cholesterol:** 0mg

26. Veggie Rolls

Preparation time: 20 minutes.

Cooking time: 20 minutes.

Servings: 5

Ingredients:

- 1 tablespoon olive oil

- 1 garlic clove, minced

- 1 teaspoon ginger, minced

- 3 scallions, chopped

- ½ pound mushrooms, chopped

- 2 cups cabbage, chopped

- 8 ounces water chestnuts, diced

- Salt and pepper to taste

- 6 spring roll wrappers

- 1 tablespoon water

Directions:

1. Add oil to a pan over medium heat.

2. Cook the garlic, ginger, scallions, and mushrooms for 2 minutes.

3. Stir in the remaining vegetables.

4. Season with salt and pepper.

5. Cook for 3 minutes, stirring.

6. Transfer to a strainer.

7. Add vegetables on top of the wrappers.

8. Roll up the wrappers.

9. Seal the edges with water.

10. Place the rolls inside the Air Fryer.

11. Choose Air Fry setting.

12. Cook at 360°F for 15 minutes.

Nutrition:

- **Calories:** 805 **Fat:** 33g **Protein:** 92g

27. Toasted Vegetables with Rice and Eggs

Preparation time: 5 minutes.

Cooking time: 13 minutes.

Servings: 4

Ingredients:

- 2 teaspoons melted butter

- 1 cup chopped mushrooms

- 1 cup cooked rice

- 1 cup peas

- 1 carrot, chopped

- 1 red onion, chopped

- 1 garlic clove, minced

- Salt and black pepper to taste

- 2 hard-boiled eggs, grated

- 1 tablespoon soy sauce

Directions:

1. Coat a baking dish with melted butter.

2. Stir together the mushrooms, carrot, peas, garlic, onion, cooked rice, salt, and pepper in a large bowl until well mixed. Pour the mixture into the prepared baking dish.

3. Place the baking dish in the Toast position.

4. Select Toast, set temperature to 380°F (193°C), and set time to 12 minutes.

5. When cooking is completed, remove from the Air Fryer grill. Divide the mixture among four plates. Serve warm with a sprinkle of grated eggs and a drizzle of soy sauce.

Nutrition:

- **Calories:** 724 **Fat:** 37g **Protein:** 62g

28. Lemony Brussels Sprouts

Preparation time: 5 minutes.

Cooking time: 19 minutes.

Servings: 4

Ingredients:

- 1 pound (454 grams) Brussels sprouts, trimmed and halved

- 1 tablespoon extra-virgin olive oil

- Sea salt and freshly ground black pepper to taste

- ½ cup sun-dried tomatoes, chopped

- 2 tablespoons freshly squeezed lemon juice

- 1 teaspoon lemon zest

Directions:

1. Line a large baking sheet with aluminum foil.

2. Toss the Brussels sprouts with olive oil in a large bowl. Sprinkle

   with salt and black pepper.

3. Spread the Brussels sprouts in a single layer on the baking sheet.

4. Place the baking sheet in the Toast position.

5. Select Toast, set temperature to 400°F (205°C), and set time to 20 minutes.

6. When done, the Brussels sprouts should be caramelized. Remove from the Air Fryer grill to a serving bowl, along with the tomatoes, lemon juice, and lemon zest. Toss to combine. Serve immediately.

Nutrition:

- **Calories:** 894

- **Fat:** 32g

- **Protein:** 92g

29. Zucchini Lasagna

Preparation time: 15 minutes.

Cooking time: 15 minutes.

Servings: 4

Ingredients:

- 1 zucchini, sliced thinly lengthwise and divided

- ½ cup marinara sauce, divided

- ¼ cup ricotta, divided

- 1 cup fresh basil leaves, chopped and divided

- ¼ cup spinach leaves, chopped and divided

Directions:

1. Layer half of the zucchini slices in a small loaf pan.

2. Spread with half of marinara sauce and ricotta.

3. Top with half of spinach and basil.

4. Repeat layers with the remaining ingredients.

5. Cover the pan with foil.

6. Place inside the Air Fryer.

7. Set it to Bake.

8. Cook at 400°F for 10 minutes.

9. Remove foil and cook for another 5 minutes.

Nutrition:

- **Calories:** 814

- **Fat:** 21g

- **Protein:** 65g

30. Eggplant Pizza

Preparation time: 25 minutes.

Cooking time: 19 minutes.

Servings: 2

Ingredients:

- 1 eggplant (sliced 1/4 -inch)

- 12 to 13 in. Gluten-free pizza dough

- ½ cup pizza sauce

- 1/4 cup fresh rosemary and basil

- ½ cup cheese 2 garlic cloves, chopped

- Red pepper, salt, and pepper to taste 1 tbsp. olive oil

Directions:

1. Rub eggplant slices with olive oil and rosemary, salt and pepper, and bake for 25 minutes at 218°C or 425°F in the Power Air Fryer Grill.

2. Roll the dough round and spread the remaining ingredients on top.

3. Preheat the Power Air Fryer Grill at 230°C or 450°F at pizza-setting and bake the pizza for 10 minutes.

Nutrition:

- **Calories:** 260

- **Protein:** 9g

- **Fat:** 14g

31. Cheesy Stuffed Mushrooms with Veggies

Preparation time: 5 minutes.

Cooking time: 9 minutes.

Servings: 4

Ingredients:

- 4 Portobello mushrooms, stem removed

- 1 tablespoon olive oil

- 1 tomato, diced

- ½ green bell pepper, diced

- ½ small red onion, diced ½ teaspoon garlic powder

- Salt and black pepper to taste ½ cup grated mozzarella cheese

Directions:

1. Using a spoon to scoop out the gills of the mushrooms and discard them. Brush the mushrooms with olive oil.

2. In a mixing bowl, stir together the remaining ingredients except for the mozzarella cheese. Using a spoon to stuff each mushroom with the filling and scatter the mozzarella cheese on top.

3. Arrange the mushrooms in the air fry basket.

4. Place the basket in the Toast position.

5. Select Toast, set temperature to 330°F (166°C), and set time to 8 minutes.

6. When cooking is completed, the cheese should be melted.

7. Serve warm.

Nutrition:

- **Calories:** 734

- **Fat:** 26g

- **Protein:** 81g

32. Toasted Mushrooms, Pepper, and Squash

Preparation time: 9 minutes.

Cooking time: 16 minutes.

Servings: 4

Ingredients:

- (8-ounces/227-grams) package sliced mushrooms

- 1 yellow summer squash, sliced

- 1 red bell pepper, sliced 2 garlic cloves, sliced

- 1 tablespoon olive oil ½ teaspoon dried basil

- ½ teaspoon dried thyme ½ teaspoon dried tarragon

Directions:

1. Toss the mushrooms, bell pepper, and squash with garlic and olive oil in a large bowl until well coated. Mix in the basil, thyme, and tarragon and toss again.

2. Spread the vegetables evenly in the air fry basket.

3. Place the basket in the Toast position.

4. Select Toast, set temperature to 350°F (180°C), and set time to 16 minutes.

5. When cooking is completed, the vegetables should be fork-tender. Remove the basket from the Air Fryer grill. Cool for 5 minutes before serving.

Nutrition:

- **Calories:** 811

- **Fat:** 30g

- **Protein:** 79g

33. Fast Lemony Wax Beans

Preparation time: 5 minutes.

Cooking time: 12 minutes.

Servings: 4

Ingredients:

- 2 pounds (907 grams) wax beans

- 2 tablespoons extra-virgin olive oil

- Salt and freshly ground black pepper to taste

- Juice of ½ lemon, for serving

Directions:

1. Line a baking sheet with aluminum foil.

2. Toss the wax beans with olive oil in a large bowl. Lightly season

   with pepper and salt.

3. Spread out the wax beans on the sheet pan.

4. Place the baking sheet in the Toast position.

5. Select Toast, set temperature to 400°F (205°C), and set time to

    12 minutes.

6. When done, the beans will be caramelized and tender. Remove

    from the Air Fryer grill to a plate and serve sprinkled with lemon

    juice.

Nutrition:

- **Calories:** 813

- **Fat:** 35g

- **Protein:** 62g

34. Sriracha Roasted Potatoes

Preparation time: 29 minutes.

Cooking time: 21 minutes.

Servings: 3

Ingredients:

- 3 potatoes, diced

- 2–3 teaspoons sriracha

- 1/4 garlic powder

- Salt & pepper to taste

- Olive oil for greasing

- Chopped fresh parsley for serving

Directions

1. Combine the potatoes with the remaining ingredients.

2. Preheat the Power Air Fryer Grill to 230°C or 450°F.

3. Line the pan with olive oil and spread the coated potatoes.

   Sprinkle parsley.

4. Bake for 30 minutes.

Nutrition:

- **Calories:** 147

- **Protein:** 3g

- **Fat:** 4.7g

Chapter 5:

Fish and Seafood Recipes

35. Baked Cajun Cod

Preparation time: 5 minutes. **Cooking time:** 12 minutes.

Servings: 2

Ingredients:

- 1 tablespoon Cajun seasoning 1 teaspoon salt

- ½ teaspoon lemon pepper

- ½ teaspoons freshly ground black pepper

- (8-ounces) cod fillets, cut to fit into the air fry basket Cooking

  spray 2 tablespoons unsalted butter, melted

- 1 lemon, cut into 4 wedges

Directions:

1. Spray the air fry basket with cooking spray.

2. Thoroughly combine the Cajun seasoning, lemon pepper, salt, and black pepper in a small bowl. Rub this mixture all over the cod fillets until completely coated.

3. Put the fillets in the Air Fry basket and brush the melted butter over both sides of each fillet.

4. Place the basket in the bake position.

5. Select Bake, set the temperature to 360°F (182°C), and set time to 12 minutes. Flip the fillets halfway through the cooking time.

6. When cooking is completed, the fish should flake apart with a fork. Remove the fillets from the Air Fryer grill and serve with fresh lemon wedges.

Nutrition:

- **Calories:** 624 **at:** 33g **Protein:** 62g

36. Crispy Salmon Patties

Preparation time: 10 minutes. **Cooking time:** 13 minutes.

Servings: 4

Ingredients:

- 1 pound salmon, chopped into ½-inch pieces

- 2 tablespoons coconut flour 2 tablespoons grated Parmesan cheese 1(½) tablespoons milk

- ½ white onion, peeled and finely chopped

- ½ teaspoon butter, at room temperature

- ½ teaspoon chipotle powder ½ teaspoon dried parsley flakes

- 1/3 teaspoon ground black pepper

- 1/3 teaspoon smoked cayenne pepper 1 teaspoon fine sea salt

Directions:

1. Put all the ingredients, except for the salmon patties in a bowl and stir to combine well.

2. Scoop out 2 tablespoons of the salmon mixture and shape into a patty with your palm, about ½ inches thick. Repeat until all the mixture is used. Transfer to the refrigerator for about 2 hours until firm.

3. When ready, arrange the salmon patties in the air fry basket.

4. Place the basket in the Bake position.

5. Select Bake, set the temperature to 395°F (202°C), and set time to 13 minutes. Flip the patties halfway through the cooking time.

6. When cooking is completed, the patties should be golden brown. Remove from the Air Fryer grill and cool for 5 minutes before serving.

Nutrition:

- **Calories:** 834

- **Fat:** 31g

- **Protein:** 62g

37. Scallops and Spring Veggies

Preparation time: 10 minutes.

Cooking time: 9 minutes.

Servings: 4

Ingredients:

- ½ pound asparagus ends trimmed, cut into 2-inch pieces

- 1 cup sugars snap peas

- 1-pound Sea scallops

- 1 tablespoon lemon juice 2 teaspoons olive oil

- ½ teaspoon dried thyme Pinch salt to taste

- Freshly ground black pepper to taste

Directions:

1. Place the asparagus and sugar snap peas in the Oven rack/basket. Place the rack on the middle-shelf of the XL Air Fryer oven.

2. Cook for 2 to 3 minutes or until the vegetables are just starting to get tender.

3. Meanwhile, check the scallops for a small muscle attached to the side, and pull it off and discard.

4. In a medium bowl, toss the scallops with lemon juice, olive oil, thyme, salt, and pepper. Place into the oven rack/basket on top of the vegetables. Place the rack on the middle-shelf of the XL Air Fryer oven.

5. Steam for 5 to 7 minutes until the scallops are just firm, and the vegetables are tender. Serve immediately.

Nutrition:

- **Calories:** 162

- **Fat:** 4g

- **Protein:** 22g

38. Tuna, Pineapple, and Grape Kebabs

Preparation time: 15 minutes.

Cooking time: 10 minutes.

Servings: 4

Ingredients:

Kebabs:

- 1 pound tuna steaks, cut into 1-inch cubes

- ½ cup large red grapes

- ½ cup canned pineapple chunks, drained, juice reserved

Marinade:

- Tablespoon honey

- 1 teaspoon olive oil

- Teaspoons grated fresh ginger

- Pinch cayenne pepper

Special Equipment:

- Metal skewers

Directions:

1. **Make the kebabs:** Thread, alternating tuna cubes, red grapes, and pineapple chunks onto the metal skewers.

2. **Make the marinade:** Whisk together the honey, olive oil, ginger, and cayenne pepper in a small bowl. Brush generously the marinade over the kebabs and allow sitting for 10 minutes.

3. When ready, transfer the kebabs to the air fry basket.

4. Place the basket in the Air Fry position.

5. Select Air Fry, set temperature to 370°F (188°C), and set time to 10 minutes.

6. After 5 minutes, remove from the Air Fryer grill and flip the kebabs and brush with the remaining marinade. Return the basket to the Air Fryer grill and continue cooking for an additional 5 minutes.

7. When cooking is completed, the kebabs should reach an internal temperature of 145°F (63°C) on a meat thermometer. Remove from the Air Fryer grill and discard any remaining marinade. Serve hot.

Nutrition:

- **Calories** 691

- **Fat** 44g

- **Protein** 80.3g

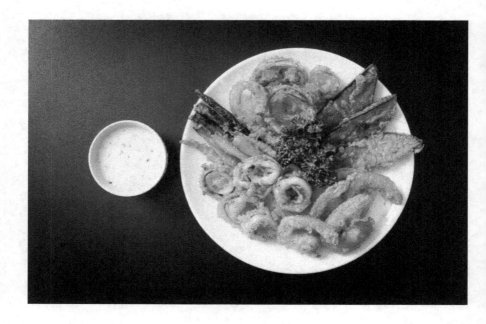

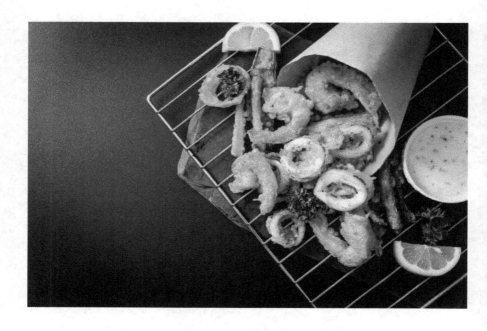

Chapter 6:

Snacks Recipes

39. Cheddar Dip

Preparation time: 5 minutes.

Cooking time: 15 minutes.

Servings: 6

Ingredients:

- 8 ounces Cheddar cheese; grated

- 12 ounces coconut cream 2 teaspoons hot sauce

Directions:

1. In a ramekin, mix the cream with hot sauce and cheese and

   whisk.

2. Put the ramekin in the fryer and cook at 390°F for 12 minutes.

Whisk, divide into bowls, and serve as a dip.

Nutrition:

- **Calories:** 170

- **Fat:** 9g

- **Fiber:** 2g

- **Carbs:** 4g

- **Protein:** 12g

Chapter 7:

Desserts Recipes

40. Cherry Pie

Preparation time: 5 minutes.

Cooking time: 25 minutes.

Servings: 8

Ingredients:

- 1 can (21 ounces) cherry pie filling

- 1 tablespoon milk

- 2 refrigerated pie crusts

- 1 egg yolk

- 1 scoop ice cream, for serving

Directions:

1. Warm the fryer at 310°F.

2. Poke holes into the crust after placing it on a pie plate. Allow the excess to hang over the edges. Place in the Air Fryer for five (5) minutes

3. Transfer the basket with the pie plate onto the countertop.

4. Fill it with the cherry filling. Remove the excess crust.

5. Cut the remaining crust into ¾-inch strips, weaving a lattice across the pie.

6. Make an egg wash using the milk and egg. Brush the pie—Air-fry for 15 minutes. Serve with a scoop of ice cream.

Nutrition:

- **Calories:** 205 **Fat:** 34g **Fiber:** 2g

- **Carbs:** 6g

- **Protein:** 2g

Conclusion

Air frying your food is one of the great alternative methods of deep-frying your food. There are various advanced Air Fryers available on the market now. In this cookbook, we have used such smart, advanced, and multifunctional cooking appliances popularly known as Power Air Fryer oven. The Power oven allows you to cook almost all types of dishes in a single cooking appliance. It is capable to cook vegetables, meat, fish, fruit slices, cakes, and more. The oven comes with different accessories, using these accessories you can cook a healthy and delicious meal at home easily. The oven is capable of roasting whole turkey or chicken at a single cooking cycle.

The Power Air Fryer is an effortless way to cook healthy and delicious foods. As a replacement for using oil, this one uses air to cook. You can cook all sorts of food, even appetizers, and snacks. Foods are cooked fast and evenly without oils. Relish cooking healthier than ever before.

The Power Air Fryer oven works on a rapid hot airflow technique which helps to distribute equally the heat into the cooking chamber around the food. This equal heat distribution cooks your food faster and gives you even cooking results in every cooking cycle. It makes your food crispy from the outside, juicy and tender from the inside. The oven comes with a big display panel with 8 preset functions. While using these preset functions, you will never be worried about temperature and time settings, as they are preset. You can also set these settings manually by pressing the up and down arrow key, pressing the up and down arrow keys given on the control panel.

This amazing appliance is simple to use. Just add the food you wish to cook and turn the 3 burners on. You can grill, fry, roast, bake, and even smoke. It can also be used to steam, boil, dehydrate and freeze. Using the Complete Power fryer, there are no limitations on what you can cook. You can also easily make healthy takeout food that would cost you a fortune.

CPSIA information can be obtained
at www.ICGtesting.com
Printed in the USA
BVHW092104240621
610373BV00002B/315